The Rowing Standard

Published by Concept Fitness
Oceanside, New York
www.conceptfitnessny.com

Paperback ISBN: 979-8-994716-0-6
eBook ISBN: 979-8-994716-1-3

Printed in the United States of America
Concept2® and Concept2 Indoor Rower® are registered trademarks of Concept2 Inc. This publication is not affiliated with or endorsed by Concept2 Inc.

First Edition - 2026 This edition reflects current coaching standards, research, and best practices at the time of publication. Future editions may include revisions, updates, or expansions as the sport and research evolve.
Version 1.0 January 2026

TABLE OF CONTENTS

INTRODUCTION

Rowing Deserves a Standard.
Rowing is one of the most effective full-body movements in fitness, yet it is often taught inconsistently, cued poorly, and rushed in environments that value intensity over technique.

That's a problem.

Good rowing isn't about pulling harder or moving faster. It's about sequence, positioning, and the ability to apply force efficiently and repeatedly without breakdown. When taught well, it builds strength, conditioning, coordination, and resilience—and the movement becomes efficient, powerful, even beautiful. Taught poorly, it becomes uncomfortable and inefficient and can ultimately lead to injury.

The widespread use of the rowing ergometer has made rowing more accessible than ever. Since the introduction of the Concept2 Indoor Rower—developed in the late 1970s by former Olympic rowers Dick and Pete Dreissigacker—rowing has expanded far beyond boathouses and competitive teams. Originally built to support high-level training, the ergometer is now used worldwide by Olympic athletes, cardiac rehabilitation patients, fitness professionals, and recreational rowers alike. Its accuracy and durability have made it the global standard for indoor rowing.

Access alone does not guarantee quality.

As rowing has entered more gyms, schools, and training environments, the movement itself has often been stripped of its technical foundation. The same machine that supports elite performance is frequently used without a shared understanding of how the stroke should look, feel, or be taught. Without a common framework, coaching becomes subjective, inconsistent, and dependent on individual interpretation rather than established principles.

This book documents the rowing standard.

Inside, you'll find clear standards for technique, common errors explained in plain language, drills that actually fix problems, and cues you can use immediately on the floor. The goal is not perfection—it's consistency. When coaches teach the same movement the same way, athletes improve faster and with fewer setbacks.

Rowing deserves that level of respect.
So do the people learning it.

CHAPTER 1: THE SCIENCE BEHIND THE STROKE

Why Rowing Works — Backed by Research

Rowing is often misunderstood.
It's labeled as "just cardio," compared casually to cycling, or dismissed as too technical to be effective for the general population. The research tells a very different story.
Decades of physiological studies show that rowing is not only safe and effective across age groups—it consistently produces greater cardiovascular demand, higher caloric expenditure, and meaningful strength engagement when compared to traditional aerobic modalities like cycling.

Let's break down the key findings from foundational rowing research and explain what they mean in real-world coaching and training.
[20-23]

1. Rowing vs. Cycling: A Fair Comparison
Multiple studies have directly compared rowing ergometry to cycling ergometry under controlled conditions—same time, similar heart rates, similar perceived effort.

What they found:
>   Heart rate feels the same
>   Effort feels the same
>   Energy demand is NOT the same

When people row and cycle at workloads they perceive as equally hard, rowing consistently requires more oxygen and burns more calories.

Key takeaway:
When effort feels equal, rowing does more.
This matters because most people self-select their training intensity. If rowing naturally demands more from the body at the same perceived effort, it becomes a more efficient and effective training tool.
[1-4]

2. Oxygen Uptake and Caloric Cost
Studies measuring VO_2 (oxygen consumption) and caloric expenditure show:
Rowing produces higher oxygen uptake than cycling at comparable heart rates. Caloric burn is significantly higher during rowing sessions. This holds true for both trained and untrained individuals

Why?

Rowing:
- Uses legs, hips, trunk, and arms
- Requires force production through large muscle groups
- Demands coordination and sequencing—not just repetition

Unlike cycling, which is primarily lower-body dominant, rowing distributes the work across the entire body.

Key takeaway: More muscle involvement = more oxygen required = higher energy cost.

2_4

3. Mechanical Efficiency and Why Technique Matters
One study examined rowing and cycling at identical power outputs.
The results showed:
- Cycling appeared mechanically "more efficient"
- Rowing required more energy to produce the same wattage

At first glance, this might seem like a negative. It isn't.

The researchers concluded that the increased energy cost in rowing is largely due to:
- Greater muscle recruitment
- Higher coordination demands
- Poor technique in inexperienced rowers

Key takeaway:
Rowing exposes inefficiency. It doesn't create it.

As technique improves, efficiency improves—but rowing will always demand more total-body involvement than cycling.

This is precisely why rowing belongs in:
- General fitness
- Athletic development
- Cardiac rehabilitation
- Aging populations

3_5

4. Rowing in Older Adults: Safe, Effective, Powerful
One of the most important findings comes from studies on elderly populations.

After 12 weeks of structured rowing training:
- VO_2 max increased significantly
- Maximum power output increased
- Cardiovascular capacity improved
- Results were comparable—or superior—to cycling

And critically:
- No increased injury risk
- Training intensities aligned with ACSM and AHA guidelines

Rowing was shown to be:
- A safe alternative
- A powerful aerobic stimulus
- Suitable even for individuals over 60

Key takeaway: This matters. Rowing isn't just for athletes. It's for longevity.
.[4-6]

5. Sub-maximal Testing: Measuring Fitness Without Maxing Out

Research on the Concept2 ergometer shows that rowing VO_2 max can be accurately estimated using sub-maximal testing—without pushing individuals to exhaustion.

At intensities of 80–90% of predicted max heart rate, VO_2 max estimates were:
- Within 5% of true values
- Highly reliable
- Practical for real-world settings

This makes rowing an excellent tool for:
- Fitness assessment
- Progress tracking
- Population-based testing
- Coaching decisions without unnecessary risk

Key takeaway: You don't have to max out to measure fitness—submaximal testing gives reliable data with far less stress on the athlete.
.[1,6]

What the Research Actually Says

Across studies, across decades, across populations:
- Rowing demands more oxygen at the same perceived effort
- Rowing burns more calories
- Rowing improves cardiovascular fitness
- Rowing builds usable strength
- Rowing scales from rehab to elite performance
- Technique matters—and improves outcomes

The science supports what good coaches already know:

Rowing is not just exercise.
It is training.

Rowing deserves a standard.

Not because it's trendy.
Not because it's hard.
Not because it looks impressive.

But because the evidence is clear:

When taught correctly, rowing is one of the most effective full-body training modalities available—capable of improving fitness, strength, efficiency, and longevity across a lifetime.

This book exists to make sure it's taught that way. [1,6]

CHAPTER 2: THE STROKE

The rowing stroke is made up of four continuous phases: **the catch, the drive, the finish, and the recovery.** While these phases are often taught separately, rowing only works when they flow together as one smooth, uninterrupted movement. Good rowing is not about "pulling" harder. It's about putting force into the machine in the correct order and allowing the body to transfer that force efficiently from the legs, through the torso, arms, and into the handle. It's actually a push, not a pull.

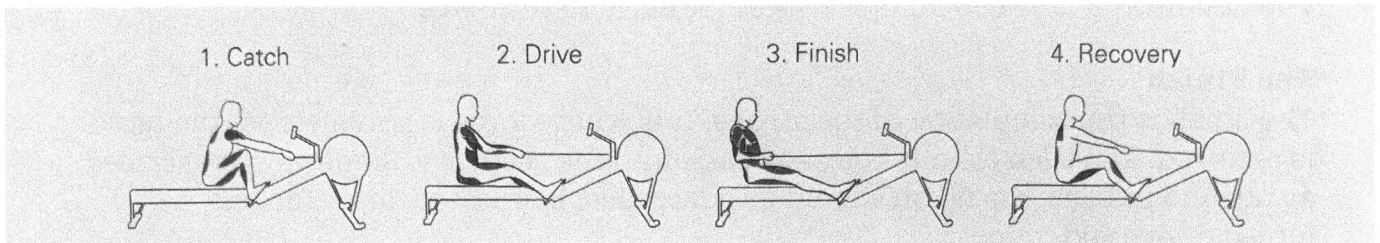

| 1. Catch | 2. Drive | 3. Finish | 4. Recovery |

Rowing is a full-body exercise, with the following breakdown of effort: 60% legs, 30% hips, and 10% arms. It's crucial to move your body from the 11 o'clock position at the catch to the 1 o'clock position at the finish, no more and no less, as deviating from this range is inefficient. There's a distinction between good length and bad length in the stroke. Leaning back too far results in bad length, while leaning to ideally 1 o'clock at the finish is considered good length, optimizing power and efficiency in each stroke. The stroke is defined by two things: length and power.

The Catch
At the catch, the rower is set up to apply power — not to create it yet.
What we want to see:
- Arms long and relaxed
- Shins close to vertical
- Chest tall, body leaning slightly forward from the hips
- Weight balanced through the feet

The catch is not about reaching as far forward as possible. Excessive forward lean or a collapsed chest puts the body in a weak position, delays power application, and can increase injury risk..

Coaching focus:
Set the position. Do not rush the next stroke.

The Drive
The drive begins with the legs and is 60% of the stroke.   The handle should move because the legs move — not the other way around.
Sequence matters:
1. Legs push
2. Body opens
3. Arms finish

If the hips open too early, leg power is lost.
If the legs extend without the body coming with them, power is delayed.

Coaching focus:
The handle and hips should move together early in the drive.

The Finish
The finish is the completion of the stroke. It is where force is transferred, the handle is received, and then cleanly released back into the recovery. Sometimes described as tap and release, the finish should be controlled, connected, and efficient—not forced or overextended.

At the finish, the power has already been produced. The goal is to receive the handle in a strong position and send it away smoothly into the next stroke.

What we want to see:

• Legs fully extended

• Torso tall with a slight lean back (approximately 100 degrees)

• Handle drawn to the sternum

• Elbows travel past the body with relaxed forearms, moving naturally—not flared wide or pinned tight.

• Wrists flat, grip light

• Shoulders down and away from the ears

The finish is not about yanking the handle or leaning excessively back. Over-pulling, shrugging the shoulders, or collapsing at the wrists disrupts flow and creates unnecessary tension. The finish should feel decisive but relaxed. The moment the handle makes contact with the body, it should be released immediately—hands move away first, then the body pivots forward, followed by the knees bending.

Coaching focus: Finish clean. Tap the body, release the handle, arms away, then pivot the body forward before approaching the catch.

The Recovery

The recovery is the reset. It is where the rower prepares the body to apply power again. While it produces no force, it determines the quality of the next stroke. A rushed or poorly sequenced recovery almost always leads to a weak catch.

The recovery begins the moment the handle leaves the body. From there, the athlete returns to the catch in a controlled, efficient order that maintains balance and posture.

Sequence matters:

1. Hands move away from the body

2. Body pivots forward from the hips

3. Knees bend and the seat rolls forward

What we want to see:

• Hands moving away smoothly and quickly

• Torso pivoting forward with the chest staying tall

• Knees remaining down until the hands clear them

• Relaxed arms and shoulders

• Controlled slide speed back to the catch

The recovery isn't passive, but it should feel calm. It sets the stage for the next powerful stroke. Rushing the slide, bending the knees too early, or collapsing the chest disrupts rhythm and makes it difficult to connect cleanly at the catch.

The recovery sets the timing of the stroke. It should be slower than the drive, a 1:2 ratio, allowing the flywheel to carry momentum while the rower regains position.

Coaching focus: Slow the slide. Set the body. Prepare to apply power.

CHAPTER 3: ROWING BASICS

Rowing performance and longevity are built on a small set of fundamental principles that govern how the athlete interfaces with the erg. Proper attire, equipment setup, and body positioning establish the conditions under which efficient force production, technical consistency, and injury prevention are possible. Errors in these foundational elements often lead to compensations that limit performance and increase strain long before faults appear in the stroke itself. Mastery of these basics ensures that every stroke begins from a position of mechanical advantage and remains repeatable across training volumes, intensities, and athlete populations.

Rowing Attire

Appropriate attire supports safe movement, efficient force transfer, and consistent technique on the rower. Clothing and footwear should allow the athlete to move freely without interfering with the stroke or the machine.

Rowers should wear:
- Comfortably fitting, nonrestrictive clothing that allows full movement at the hips, knees, ankles, and shoulders
- Clothing that does not hang below the seat, reducing the risk of fabric catching in the seat rollers
- Footwear that allows complete flexion and extension of the ankle joint while providing a stable platform for force application

Footwear Selection

Flat-soled athletic shoes are preferred over cushioned running shoes for rowing. Running shoes are designed to absorb impact and compress under load. While this cushioning is beneficial for running, it is counterproductive on the rowing machine.

A soft or "squishy" sole reduces the athlete's ability to push effectively through the foot stretcher. Instead of force being transferred directly into the flywheel, some energy is lost as the shoe compresses. This compromises power application, delays connection at the catch, and can alter lower-body mechanics.

Flat-soled shoes provide a firm, stable foundation that allows the rower to push cleanly through the heels and mid-foot. This improves force transfer, enhances consistency in the drive, and reduces unnecessary movement at the ankle. A stable shoe helps the athlete feel grounded, balanced, and connected to the machine.

Coaching focus:
Stable feet create a stable stroke. Choose footwear that supports force transfer, not impact absorption.

Foot Stretcher Setting

Adjust the foot stretcher according to your shoe size so that the black strap lines up with the widest part of your foot—typically around your first set of shoelaces. This ensures optimal leg drive and ankle mobility throughout the stroke.

Quick Release Technique

To quickly release your feet from the foot stretchers, press down on the clips while lifting your toes upward. Then, point your toes down and kick your feet up and out. Practice this a few times—it's a key move in both training and racing.

Seated Position

Your sitting position on the erg is critical for power transfer and long-term comfort. Sit directly on your sit bones, not rolled under on your lower back. The center of your pelvis (your "taint") should be in the middle of the seat, allowing your body to pivot freely. At the catch position, your hamstrings should be in light contact with your seat. This position sets you up for a powerful and safe stroke sequence.

Hand Placement on the Handle

Hold the handle like you're holding two small birds—firm enough so they don't fly away, but loose enough so you don't crush them. Keep your hands relaxed, with your fingers gently wrapped around the handle. Thumbs should wrap underneath and around the handle. Avoid choking up on the handle or letting your wrists bend or collapse. Your wrist is an extension of the stroke. Proper grip helps you maintain clean technique and reduces fatigue in longer sessions.

Performance Monitor Positioning for Taller Athletes

For taller rowers, monitor height matters. On the Concept2 PM5 (or similar performance monitors), the screen can be easily adjusted to suit your line of sight and posture.

If you're a taller athlete, raise the monitor arm so the screen sits higher and more upright. This small adjustment allows you to maintain better posture, especially at the catch position, where taller rowers often round forward to see the screen.

A properly positioned monitor helps you:

- Keep your chest lifted and spine long

- Avoid unnecessary strain on your neck and upper back

- Maintain consistent eye level without dropping your head

This is a simple, often overlooked fix that makes a big difference in comfort, performance, and technique — especially in longer sessions or high-intensity intervals.

CHAPTER 4: COMMON WARM-UPS FOR ROWING SESSIONS

A solid warm-up prepares rowers both mentally and physically for practice. No athlete ever outgrows the basics—warm-ups are not just preparation, they are skill development. Below are drills we regularly use to get ready for training.

1. Pick Drill (Technique-Focused Warm-Up)
A progressive drill that breaks down the rowing stroke into components to reinforce body awareness and sequencing.

Progression Example:

Arms Only – Focus on clean finish and controlled hands-away.

Body and Arms Only – Add the hip swing, moving the torso like the hands of a clock from 11 to 1, while keeping the legs straight.

Legs Only – Drive from the legs without using arms or body swing. Full Stroke – Put it all together with clean transitions.

2. Pause Drills
Helps rowers develop control and refine stroke timing. Arms away (pause), body forward (pause), stroke.

3. Power 10
A burst of 10 strokes with maximal pressure and focus. Used to prime the body for harder work. Power is generally built through a series of 3 power 10s.

4. Drill Combinations (Approx. 3 Minutes)
Warm-ups often include combinations of the above to build rhythm and reinforce technique:
Example Sequence (approx. 3 minutes):
- 10 strokes Arms Only
- 10 strokes Body & Arms
- 10 strokes at pause drill
- Power 10 x3
- Stroke build (see below)

5. Stroke Rate Build (Rate Ladders)
Used to gradually elevate heart rate and sharpen timing before the main workout.
Stroke Build:
10 strokes at each: 22, 24, 26, 28, 30 SPM

Option: spend 1 min or 30 seconds at each rate instead of stroke count
Focus on maintaining technique as rate increases

6. Strapless Rowing / Drills

Rowing without foot straps and sometimes even without the handle can promote core stability, balance, and proper connection to the machine. Strapless rowing reinforces correct sequencing and prevents athletes from relying on the straps for power or control.

Strapless Body Positioning Drills:
• Arms out straight, maintaining body position between 11 o'clock and 1 o'clock
• Arms to the head, holding 11–1 o'clock posture
• Arms overhead, maintaining 11–1 o'clock body angle
• Legs and hips only (no handle), focusing on controlled drive and recovery

These drills develop body awareness, balance, and efficient movement through the stroke.

7. On-Erg Stretching

Incorporate mobility work before or after warm-up to enhance range of motion and prevent injury.
Examples:
Hamstring Stretch – One foot out of the foot stretcher, reach forward.
Seated Windmill – Rotate upper body side to side with arm extension.
Open Book Stretch – open arms wide in a twisting motion.
Taylor Stretch – cross one leg over the other. Gentle pressure on the upper knee, lean forward for hip mobility.

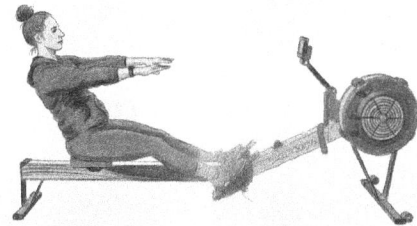

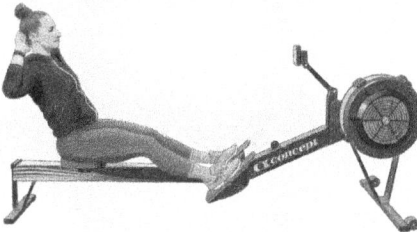

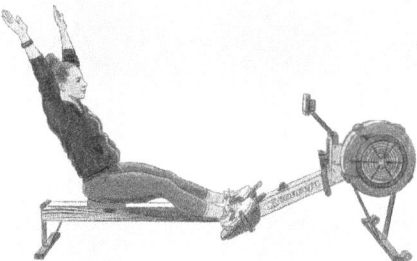

Form - Power - Speed

Form takes precedence over power and speed.
Without proper form, power is unattainable, and without power, speed is unachievable. When all elements align, magic occurs. After mastering form, power is dictated by the force exerted during the catch and drive phases of the stroke. Speed is determined by the rate at which you return to the catch position. Coach this relentlessly.

CHAPTER 5: ADAPTATIONS

Rowing is a full-body movement that, when performed with proper technique, can help build strength and resilience. However, injuries and physical limitations may require adjustments to your form or training approach.

Technique Modifications for Injury or Limitation
Learn how to adapt the rowing stroke to accommodate common injuries or conditions:

Ankle injuries or limited mobility: Shorten the compression at the catch to reduce stress on the joint.

Knee injuries: Limit knee bend and prioritize a controlled, deliberate leg drive. Use a more upright position to reduce stress on the joint. If needed, modify the workout to body-and-arms rowing only, keeping the legs straight.

Back injuries: Minimize layback and avoid excessive hinging at the hips. Maintain a neutral spine throughout the stroke.

Pregnancy: Reduce intensity and range of motion, keeping movements controlled. Prioritize core stability and breathing over power.

Understanding how to safely adjust the rowing stroke can allow athletes to continue training while protecting injured or vulnerable areas.

CHAPTER 6: STRENGTH TRAINING FOR INJURY PREVENTION

Before we talk about rowing more, we need to talk about durability. A well-rounded strength training program is not optional for rowers—it is foundational. Rowing is a high-repetition, high-force sport that places significant demands on the hips, spine, and shoulders. Without adequate strength, these repeated forces are absorbed by passive structures like joints, ligaments, and discs instead of the muscles designed to handle load, leading over time to overuse injuries. As supported by the research discussed earlier on older adult rowers, appropriately prescribed resistance training is safe and protective. This does not require maximal or aggressive loading; instead, strength training should prioritize sound movement, progressive overload, and recovery to build durability, preserve joint health, and support long-term performance across all ages.

Strength training builds the armor that protects a rower's body. The goal is not to "lift heavy for the sake of lifting," but to develop resilient, balanced athletes who can produce force safely and repeatedly. Strength training builds resilience.

Key foundational movements include:

- Deadlift – develops the posterior chain (glutes, hamstrings, spinal stabilizers), teaching athletes to hinge correctly and protect the lower back during the drive.

- Squat – builds leg strength and reinforces proper knee, hip, and ankle mechanics that transfer directly to powerful leg drive.

- Clean and Press – trains coordinated power from the legs through the core to the upper body, reinforcing full-body sequencing and force transfer.

- Pull-ups – strengthen the lats, upper back, and grip, supporting posture and shoulder health through the finish and recovery.

- Push-ups – balance the upper body, develop shoulder stability, and protect against imbalances created by repetitive pulling.

- Planks – train core stiffness and endurance, allowing the athlete to transmit force efficiently without collapsing through the spine.

Together, these movements create a strong posterior chain, a stable and responsive core, and balanced upper-body strength. This reduces unnecessary stress on the spine and shoulders, improves power output, and significantly lowers injury risk—especially during high-volume training phases.

CHAPTER 7: MOBILITY FOR PERFORMANCE AND LONGEVITY

Strength alone is not enough. Mobility is what allows strength to be expressed effectively and safely on the erg and on the water.

Rowing demands repeated movement through deep hip and ankle ranges. When mobility is limited, the body compensates—often at the lumbar spine or shoulders—leading to inefficient movement patterns and increased injury risk. Mobility work ensures that rowers can access the positions required for proper technique without forcing them.

Ankle and hip mobility are especially critical for:

• Achieving a strong, balanced catch position

• Maintaining proper shin angle and posture

• Allowing the hips to do the work instead of the lower back

• Supporting smooth, controlled recovery and clean sequencing

Regular mobility training improves range of motion, enhances movement quality, and reduces joint strain. Just as importantly, it allows athletes to continue rowing well into adulthood. Longevity in the sport depends on preserving joint health, maintaining tissue quality, and avoiding the accumulation of small movement faults over thousands of strokes.

When strength and mobility are trained together, rowers move better, produce more power with less effort, and stay healthier over the long term. This is not supplemental work—it is part of the rowing standard. Mobility preserves access to key positions.

CHAPTER 8: COMMON ROWING INJURIES

Rowing is a repetitive, high-load sport. While technically low impact, the accumulation of force over thousands of strokes places consistent stress on the same joints and tissues. Most rowing injuries are not the result of a single traumatic event, but rather small technical faults, strength deficits, or mobility restrictions compounded over time.

Understanding common rowing injuries—and how to address them through intelligent training—allows athletes to stay healthy, return to rowing faster, and continue progressing even during periods of modified work.

Lower Back Pain and Lumbar Strain

Why it happens: Lower back pain is the most common rowing complaint. It often stems from poor hip hinge mechanics, limited hip mobility, weak glutes, or an inability to maintain trunk stiffness during the drive. When the hips cannot generate force effectively, the lumbar spine compensates—absorbing load it was never designed to handle repeatedly.

What needs to be strengthened:
- Glutes and hamstrings
- Deep core stabilizers
- Posterior chain endurance
- Hip hinge mechanics

What needs mobility work:
- Hips (especially flexion and internal rotation)
- Ankles (to allow proper catch position without lumbar flexion)

Rehab and return-to-rowing movements:
- Romanian deadlifts (light to moderate, controlled)
- Hip bridges and hip thrusts
- Dead bugs and side planks
- Goblet squats emphasizing posture
- Tempo rowing drills with reduced range (when appropriate)

The goal is restoring force production at the hips while maintaining a neutral, stable spine under load.

Elbow Pain / "Tennis Elbow" (Lateral Epicondylitis)

Why it happens:
Elbow pain in rowers is commonly caused by excessive grip tension, overuse of the forearms, and poor sequencing that shifts work away from the legs and lats. Athletes who "pull early" or over-grip the handle place constant strain on the elbow extensors.

What needs to be strengthened:
- Forearm extensors (eccentrically)
- Upper back and lats
- Grip endurance without excessive tension

What needs to be addressed technically:
- Relaxed hands
- Proper leg-driven sequencing
- Lat engagement over arm dominance

Rehab and return-to-rowing movements:
- Eccentric wrist extension exercises
- Supported rows focusing on lat engagement
- Strapless rowing drills to reduce grip dependency
- Banded pull-downs with relaxed hands
- Push-ups to rebalance upper-body loading

Reducing grip tension while improving force transfer through the larger muscle groups is key to recovery.

Rib Stress Fractures
Why they happen:
Rib stress fractures are common in competitive rowers, particularly during periods of high volume or rapid training increases. They are often linked to poor trunk stability, excessive layback, asymmetrical force application, or fatigue that leads to loss of control at the finish.

What needs to be strengthened:
- Trunk stabilizers (especially anti-rotation)
- Serratus anterior and upper back
- Breathing mechanics under load

What needs to be limited initially:
- High stroke rate
- Aggressive layback
- Long sessions on the erg

Rehab and return-to-rowing movements:
- Pallof presses and cable anti-rotation holds
- Controlled rowing arms-only and body-over drills
- Light rowing at low rates once pain-free
- Push-up plus variations for scapular control
- Gradual reintroduction of full strokes

Return must be gradual, respecting tissue healing timelines while maintaining overall conditioning.

Shoulder Pain and Impingement

Why it happens:
Shoulder pain often results from muscular imbalance—strong pulling muscles without adequate scapular control or pressing balance. Poor posture, rounded shoulders, and fatigue at the finish exacerbate the issue.

What needs to be strengthened:
- Scapular stabilizers
- Rotator cuff
- Balanced pushing patterns

Rehab and return-to-rowing movements:
- Scapular push-ups
- Face pulls and banded external rotation
- Bottom-up kettlebell carries
- Push-ups with controlled tempo
- Reduced layback and clean handle paths on the erg

Healthy shoulders depend on balanced strength and consistent positioning. Intelligent rehab keeps athletes moving forward instead of starting over. Incorporating the crossover symmetry system into warmups is a great tool to keep shoulders healthy.

CHAPTER 9: TRAINING THROUGH INJURY: MAINTAINING FITNESS WITHOUT LOSING PROGRESS

Being sidelined from rowing does not mean being sidelined from training.

Injured rowers regularly use the C2 bike as a primary conditioning tool during periods when rowing volume must be reduced or eliminated. Cycling allows athletes to maintain aerobic capacity, leg strength, and mental engagement without the repetitive spinal and upper-body loading of the erg.

Bike sessions are programmed intentionally to:
- Preserve endurance
- Maintain training structure
- Reduce frustration during rehab periods
- Enable a smoother transition back to rowing

By continuing to train intelligently, athletes return to the rower fitter, more resilient, and less likely to re-injure themselves. Intelligent rehab keeps athletes moving forward instead of starting over.
Rowers deserve a system that keeps them rowing, not just this season, but for decades.[20-23]

CHAPTER 10: BREATHING TECHNIQUES

Power comes from mechanics. Mechanics depend on breathing. Breathing is a foundational yet often overlooked component of rowing performance. Efficient breathing supports power production, endurance, posture, and overall movement quality. In a sport where athletes repeatedly produce force while maintaining precise sequencing, breathing must work with the stroke—not against it.

Many rowers naturally synchronize their breathing with the rhythm of the stroke. A common and effective pattern is to exhale during the drive, when force output is highest, and inhale during the recovery as the body returns to the catch. This pattern supports trunk stability, reduces unnecessary tension, and allows for sustained effort over longer pieces.

That said, breathing patterns are not one-size-fits-all. Athletes should experiment within training to find a rhythm that allows them to remain relaxed, powerful, and efficient. The goal is consistent airflow. Breath holding, particularly during high-effort strokes, increases internal pressure, limits oxygen delivery, and often leads to early fatigue or breakdown in technique.

There has also been growing interest in nasal breathing and other breathing strategies during low- to moderate-intensity training. Some studies suggest potential benefits related to aerobic efficiency, respiratory control, and perceived exertion. While these methods may have value in specific contexts, they should never compromise stroke quality or output. Breathing strategies are tools—not rules—and must always serve the demands of the session.

Research Context and Breathing Strategies

Research in endurance sport and rowing biomechanics consistently demonstrates that breathing influences trunk stability, oxygen delivery, and fatigue management. Studies examining both ergometer and on-water rowing show that coordinated breathing patterns can reduce unnecessary muscular tension, improve movement efficiency, and delay respiratory fatigue—particularly during steady-state and longer-duration work.

Additional research focusing on masters and older athletes highlights the role of controlled breathing in supporting postural control and reducing excessive spinal loading during repeated force production. This reinforces the importance of breathing not only for performance, but also for longevity in the sport.

More recent investigations have explored nasal breathing, respiratory muscle training, and cadence-based breathing during aerobic training. These approaches suggest potential improvements in ventilatory efficiency, carbon dioxide tolerance, and perceived exertion during low- to moderate-intensity efforts. However, the research is equally clear that breathing strategies must match the technical and metabolic demands of the session. Techniques that restrict airflow or disrupt rhythm may be useful as training tools, but they are not appropriate during high-power or race-pace rowing.

In short, breathing strategies should enhance stroke quality—not override it.

Common Breathing Techniques in Rowing
Drive-Exhale / Recovery-Inhale
This is the most commonly observed and often most effective breathing pattern in rowing. Exhaling during the drive supports trunk stiffness and force transfer through the legs and hips, while inhaling during the recovery allows the athlete to relax, reset posture, and prepare for the next catch.

Two-Stroke Breathing (Endurance Pieces)
During longer steady-state work, some athletes naturally shift to breathing every two strokes. This can help regulate effort and prevent breath holding, provided it remains relaxed and unforced.

Free Breathing (High-Rate or Race Pace)
At high stroke rates or maximal efforts, breathing may decouple from the stroke entirely. This is normal and often necessary. In these situations, continuous airflow takes priority over precise timing.

Nasal Breathing (Low-Intensity Training Only)
Nasal breathing may be used selectively during warm-ups or aerobic base work to encourage diaphragmatic breathing and relaxation. If nasal breathing alters stroke mechanics, posture, or power output, it should be abandoned immediately.

Breathing Drills for Rowers
Breath Awareness Rows
Row at low intensity and consciously pair exhale with the drive for 10–15 strokes at a time. The goal is awareness and relaxation, not perfection.

Silent Drive Drill
During steady rowing, focus on a smooth, quiet exhale through the drive phase. This helps reduce excessive bracing and tension in the neck and shoulders.

Pause Drill with Breathing Control
Use pause rowing at arms-away or body-over positions while maintaining calm nasal or controlled mouth breathing. This reinforces relaxed breathing during technically demanding positions.

Warm-Up Nasal Breathing
During the first 5–10 minutes of warm-up, nasal breathing can promote relaxation and diaphragmatic engagement before transitioning to unrestricted breathing as intensity increases.

Off-Erg Diaphragmatic Breathing
Supine or seated breathing drills outside of rowing help athletes learn to expand the rib cage and abdomen without excessive spinal movement or bracing, reinforcing efficient breathing mechanics that transfer back to the stroke.

Coaching Takeaway
Breathing should support rhythm, posture, and force—not compete with them. The most effective breathing pattern is the one that allows the athlete to remain relaxed under load, maintain technical consistency, and sustain effort across the demands of training and racing. Coaches should treat breathing as a skill: introduce it in low-pressure settings, reinforce it during technical work, and allow it to adapt naturally as intensity rises.

Above all, effective rowing requires continuous, controlled breathing. Athletes who breathe well move better, last longer, and maintain technical integrity deeper into training and racing. Simply put: breathe early, breathe often, and never let breathing become a limiter to performance. [20-21]

CHAPTER 11: USING THE ROWING MONITOR

Why the Monitor Matters

The Performance Monitor is what makes Concept2 different from every other rowing machine on the market. It's not just a screen—it's your truth-teller, your scoreboard, and, when used correctly, one of your best coaching tools. The monitor allows you to train with intention instead of just "paddling."

Every number on the screen tells a story:

- **Split time** reflects pace and consistency

- **Stroke rate** reveals efficiency and rhythm

- **Watts and calories** reflect power output

- **Heart rate** (when connected) shows internal workload and recovery

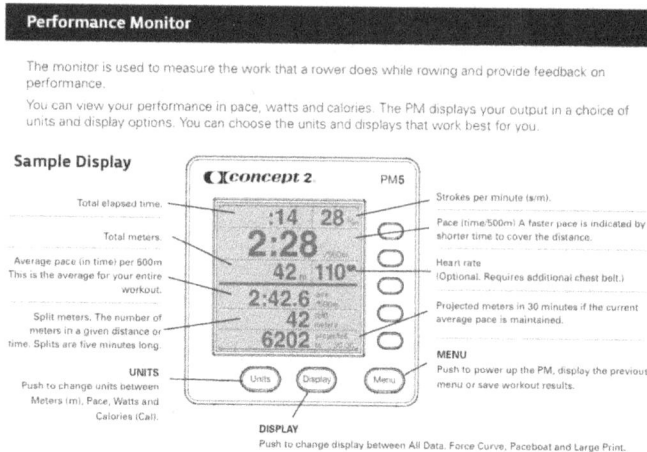

Performance Monitor

The monitor is used to measure the work that a rower does while rowing and provide feedback on performance.

You can view your performance in pace, watts and calories. The PM displays your output in a choice of units and display options. You can choose the units and displays that work best for you.

This isn't about competing with others. It's you versus you. The monitor keeps training honest, focused, and measurable—turning effort into information.

At its core, the monitor measures the work performed on each stroke. The flywheel responds directly to how much force you apply, and the monitor converts that force into readable data. When understood properly, this data reinforces good technique, smarter pacing, and long-term progress.

Performance Metrics and Training Concepts

The Concept2 Performance Monitor displays rowing output using three primary metrics: **calories, meters, and watts**. Each represents the same underlying work, simply expressed in different units. Understanding what each metric means—and how to use it—prevents common training mistakes and improves efficiency.

Calories vs. Meters vs. Watts

Calories

Calories represent estimated energy expenditure. While calories are a popular metric because they feel simple and relatable, the rowing machine does not directly measure calories burned. Instead, calories are calculated from power output using an estimation model.

Rowing for calories does not require a different technique than rowing for meters or watts. Altering technique to "chase calories" often results in inefficiency and longer completion times. Technique should remain consistent regardless of the metric chosen.

Meters

Meters indicate the distance rowed based on flywheel movement and stroke length. Distance-based rowing is commonly paired with split times, measured as time per 500 meters. Split time is the most widely used performance metric in rowing and provides a clear indicator of pacing and consistency.

Meters and splits are ideal for endurance training, benchmarking, and long-term progress tracking.

Watts

Watts measure power output—the rate at which work is performed. This metric responds immediately to changes in force application and is unaffected by stroke rate or drag factor. Because of this, watts are often the most honest indicator of effort.

Watts are especially useful for technical work, strength-focused sessions, and teaching athletes how to apply force efficiently rather than simply rowing faster.

While calories, meters, and watts all describe the same work, watts tell you how the work is being produced, splits tell you how fast, and calories estimate how costly it is to the body.

Understanding Pace, Power, and Efficiency

Pace and power are directly related—but not linearly. Small improvements in split time require disproportionately large increases in power output. This explains why dropping even one second off a split becomes increasingly difficult at higher levels. This relationship reinforces an essential rowing principle: efficiency matters more than effort. Better sequencing, posture, and timing allow athletes to generate more power with less fatigue.

Stroke Output and Consistency

The monitor also displays stroke output, which reflects the amount of work produced on the most recent stroke. Inconsistent stroke output often signals rushed recoveries, poor sequencing, or breakdowns in posture.

Developing rowers tend to chase pace, while skilled rowers learn to control stroke output. Over time, consistent output becomes a stronger indicator of proficiency than raw speed alone.

Stroke Rate (SPM)

Stroke rate, displayed as strokes per minute (SPM), reflects how frequently the athlete takes a stroke—not how hard they pull. Stroke rate is primarily influenced by the speed of the recovery phase.

Higher stroke rates without increased power simply spin the flywheel faster without producing more work per stroke. Athletes often feel like they're working harder, but without added force, the extra rate doesn't translate to greater output. Effective rowing balances rate and power—using lower rates to build strength and precision, and higher rates for racing and high-intensity efforts.

Using the Monitor Intentionally

The Performance Monitor does not force intensity—it reflects it. Athletes choose how much effort to apply, and the monitor reports the result. This makes it a powerful teaching tool when paired with coaching and technical awareness.

Tracking and Performance Accountability

Consistent performance tracking is a fundamental component of effective rowing training. Objective data collected from the rowing monitor allows athletes and coaches to evaluate pacing, efficiency, and progress over time. Without systematic tracking, improvements are difficult to verify and training decisions become subjective rather than evidence-based.

If athletes aren't using a training app like ErgZone or ErgData, they should take a photo of the monitor at the end of each workout and save it to their phone. Over time, this creates a personal performance archive that documents pacing, splits, consistency, and progress. This simple habit builds accountability, improves self-awareness, and supports smarter goal setting from session to session. Track it, or it didn't happen.

While the official Concept2 apps (ErgData and ErgZone) provide seamless integration and reliable logging, many rowers and coaches also use third-party platforms such as MyRow, RowPro, LiveRowing, and PainSled for deeper analytics, expanded workout libraries, or social tracking. The specific tool matters less than the habit itself; the right platform is the one that supports the athlete's goals—whether that's pacing discipline, physiological monitoring, long-term trend analysis, or community engagement.

Workout Types to Know

Understanding how to properly set up workouts on the Performance Monitor ensures consistency and accurate data collection.

Single Distance

Used for fixed-distance rows such as 2K, 5K, or 10K efforts. Ideal for testing, pacing practice, and uninterrupted work.

Single Time

Used for continuous rowing over a set duration (e.g., 20–60 minutes). Commonly used for aerobic development and Zone 2 (UT2) training.

Single Calories

Used to row continuously until a calorie target is reached. Common in conditioning workouts, while still requiring the same technical standards.

Undefined Rest

Used when rest periods are variable or athletes are rotating on and off the machine. Common in class-based or partner workouts. Note: this setting does not allow for re-row.

Intervals – Meters

Distance-based intervals with programmed rest. Ideal for race-pace work, threshold training, and repeatability under fatigue.

Intervals – Time

Time-based intervals with structured rest. Useful for aerobic power, pacing discipline, and consistency.

Intervals – Calories

Calorie-based intervals with programmed rest. Popular in group settings while still demanding technical precision.

Variable Intervals

Custom combinations of distance, time, and calories. Best suited for advanced programming and competition-style workouts.

Coaching Takeaway

The rowing monitor is a mirror—not a motivator. It reflects how well force is applied through sound movement and controlled rhythm. When used correctly, it supports technique, reinforces pacing discipline, and tracks progress over time.

Chasing numbers at the expense of posture, sequencing, or breathing undermines long-term development. Master the stroke first. Let the numbers follow.

CHAPTER 12: DRAG FACTOR

Drag factor is a pivotal concept in rowing because it directly influences how the stroke feels to the athlete. It represents the amount of wind resistance applied to the flywheel and determines how much load the athlete feels at the catch. Drag factor is controlled by the damper on the side of the flywheel, but the damper setting itself is only a lever—not the measurement. The true value is the drag factor number, which can be viewed on the Performance Monitor by navigating to Menu → More Options → Display Drag Factor and beginning to row.

Adjusting the damper changes how much air is allowed into the flywheel, thereby increasing or decreasing drag factor. A higher drag factor creates a heavier feel at the catch and requires more force to accelerate the flywheel, while a lower drag factor demands cleaner sequencing and a stronger connection to the machine without relying on wind resistance for feedback.

A common misconception is that stronger athletes should row with the damper set to 10. In reality, most elite and Olympic-level rowers use relatively low damper settings—typically around 3 to 6—corresponding to a drag factor between approximately 115 and 130, depending on the duration of the piece and the size of the athlete. Strength alone does not justify a higher drag; technical proficiency, efficiency, and rhythm are far more important determinants of performance.

Drag Factor and Catch Quality
Drag factor can be a valuable coaching tool for developing and assessing the quality of the catch. A technically sound catch—characterized by proper body position, early connection, and effective force transfer—allows an athlete to row efficiently at lower drag factors. Athletes with a strong, connected catch often feel no need for excessive resistance from the machine.

When the chain fails to engage smoothly at the catch—resulting in a slipping or delayed connection—a slightly higher drag factor may provide clearer tactile feedback and help the athlete feel the moment of engagement. Conversely, when the stroke appears to devolve into a "tug-of-war" between the athlete and the flywheel—where force application is abrupt, heavy, or disconnected—the drag factor is often too high and should be reduced. Excessive drag can cause technical flaws, encourage over-bracing, and disrupt rhythm.

The goal is not to use drag factor to compensate for poor mechanics, but to use it strategically to expose and refine them.

Consistency and Individualization
Maintaining a consistent drag factor is essential for meaningful performance tracking. When drag factor remains stable, changes in split times, watts, and stroke

efficiency can be attributed to improvements in fitness or technique rather than changes in machine resistance. This consistency also ensures a comparable training experience across different ergs and locations.

Optimal drag factor varies between athletes based on strength, technical skill, and training objectives. Experimentation during training can help athletes identify appropriate settings for different types of work. One effective method is a damper progression test, such as five rounds of 20 seconds on and 20 seconds off, gradually adjusting the damper from 2 through 10 while monitoring drag factor and stroke feel. This allows athletes to experience how wind resistance influences connection, rhythm, and fatigue.

Applying Drag Factor to Training

Drag factor may be adjusted according to workout type or training phase. Lower drag factors are generally better suited for longer steady-state rows, technical work, and aerobic development. Higher drag factors may be appropriate for short, high-intensity intervals or specific strength-focused sessions, provided the athlete's technique can support the increased load without degradation.

Quick Reference: Drag Factor Guidelines

Training Context	Typical Drag Factor Range	Purpose / Notes
Technical Drills & Skill Work	100–110	Promotes clean sequencing and exposes connection errors
Long Steady-State (UT2 / Zone 2)	105–115	Encourages efficiency, rhythm, and sustainable effort
General Training / Mixed Work	110–120	Balanced resistance for most sessions
Race-Pace & Threshold Work	115–125	Allows strong connection without excessive load
Short Power Intervals	120–130	Used selectively for strength emphasis; technique must be solid
Advanced / Elite Rowers	110–118	Most elite athletes stay within this range year-round
Masters / Older Athletes	100–115	Reduces joint and spinal strain while maintaining stroke quality

Note: Adjust ranges based on technique quality and individual response.

Ultimately, drag factor should enhance stroke quality—not overpower it. When set correctly, it reinforces proper sequencing, promotes an effective catch, and supports sustainable, repeatable rowing.

14–16

CHAPTER 13: RACING & PACING

The 2K
Dive into the significance of this challenging test and its impact on our training regimen:

1. Importance: The 2000m test isn't just a fitness benchmark; it's a vital gauge of our endurance, strength, and mental resilience. It sets the tone for performance improvement and goal setting. The pace we hold becomes our new first name. It becomes part of your identity as an athlete.

2. Pacing : After completing the 2k test, we learn pacing we can use for all our training moving forward. 2k + 12 to 20 on longer intervals and 2k + 2 to -2 on sprint intervals. Allowing for negative splits and increasing our aerobic capacity in the most efficient way. It's our ultimate litmus test, guiding us on how to pace every aspect of our training sessions, ensuring optimal effort and efficiency.

3. The Journey: the 2K test demands everything you've got - physical power, mental fortitude, and strategic execution. It's a rollercoaster of emotions, pushing your limits with every stroke. We start with the sprint start (8 insanely fast strokes.) Settle in to the race pace. Hang on for dear life through that third 500 and then finish strong. Prepare yourself for the discomfort so it doesn't come as a shock when it hits. Welcome the pain. It means you're doing it right. Get comfortable being uncomfortable.

4. Post-Test Triumph: When executed flawlessly, the feeling post-2000m is unmatched. It's a cocktail of accomplishment, pride, and the sweet taste of progress. Sometimes a breathless cough. You've conquered the challenge and emerged stronger than ever.

5. Mind Games: Let's not overlook the psychology at play. The 2K test is as much a battle of the mind as it is of the body. It's about silencing the inner doubts, staying focused, and pushing through the discomfort zone.
Embrace the grind, feel the burn, and conquer the 2000m - because greatness awaits beyond the finish line.
This is the ultimate test. If you're interested in rowing on a collegiate level this is one of the major components coaches will be looking at.

Pacing Strategies
Understanding pacing is key to long-term performance and injury prevention. One of the most useful strategies we teach is the "feels like 2K+5" rule — meaning you row at a pace that feels 5 seconds slower per 500m than your 2K race pace. This creates a mental anchor for effort and intensity during workouts.

Pacing for Time Trials

Time trials demand discipline more than bravery. The goal is not to row the fastest possible first 500 meters, but to row the fastest average pace you can sustain without technical breakdown.

In a 2K, early overpacing leads to rapid fatigue and compromised sequencing long before the finish. Athletes should aim to feel controlled in the first half, allowing effort to build gradually rather than spike early. For longer efforts such as a 5K, pacing must feel almost restrained at the start, with consistency taking priority over aggression.

Effective time-trial pacing preserves posture, breathing, and rhythm so that speed is maintained—not forced—throughout the piece.

Pacing in Mixed-Modality Workouts

In mixed-modality training, pacing is often misunderstood. Athletes frequently row too hard early, compromising performance on subsequent movements. The row should support the workout—not sabotage it.

		Concept2 Indoor Rower Pace Chart					
	Use this chart to predict your final time or distance for the workouts shown.						
Average pace per	Your time will be:					Your distance will be:	
500m	1000m	2000m	5000m	6000m	10,000m	30 min.	60 min.
1:40	3:20	6:40	16:40	20:00	33:20	9000	18,000
1:42	3:24	6:48	17:00	20:24	34:00	8824	17,647
1:44	3:28	6:56	17:20	20:48	34:40	8654	17,308
1:46	3:32	7:04	17:40	21:12	35:20	8491	16,981
1:48	3:36	7:12	18:00	21:36	36:00	8333	16,667
1:50	3:40	7:20	18:20	22:00	36:40	8182	16,364
1:52	3:44	7:28	18:40	22:24	37:20	8036	16,071
1:54	3:48	7:36	19:00	22:48	38:00	7895	15,789
1:56	3:52	7:44	19:20	23:12	38:40	7759	15,517
1:58	3:56	7:52	19:40	23:36	39:20	7627	15,254
2:00	4:00	8:00	20:00	24:00	40:00	7500	15,000
2:02	4:04	8:08	20:20	24:24	40:40	7377	14,754
2:04	4:08	8:16	20:40	24:48	41:20	7258	14,516
2:06	4:12	8:24	21:00	25:12	42:00	7143	14,286
2:08	4:16	8:32	21:20	25:36	42:40	7031	14,063
2:10	4:20	8:40	21:40	26:00	43:20	6923	13,846
2:12	4:24	8:48	22:00	26:24	44:00	6818	13,636
2:14	4:28	8:56	22:20	26:48	44:40	6716	13,433
2:16	4:32	9:04	22:40	27:12	45:20	6618	13,235
2:18	4:36	9:12	23:00	27:36	46:00	6522	13,043
2:20	4:40	9:20	23:20	28:00	46:40	6429	12,857
2:22	4:44	9:28	23:40	28:24	47:20	6338	12,676
2:24	4:48	9:36	24:00	28:48	48:00	6250	12,500
2:26	4:52	9:44	24:20	29:12	48:40	6164	12,329
2:28	4:56	9:52	24:40	29:36	49:20	6081	12,162
2:30	5:00	10:00	25:00	30:00	50:00	6000	12,000
2:32	5:04	10:08	25:20	30:24	50:40	5921	11,842
2:34	5:08	10:16	25:40	30:48	51:20	5844	11,688
2:36	5:12	10:24	26:00	31:12	52:00	5769	11,538
2:38	5:16	10:32	26:20	31:36	52:40	5696	11,392
2:40	5:20	10:40	26:40	32:00	53:20	5625	11,250
2:42	5:24	10:48	27:00	32:24	54:00	5556	11,111
2:44	5:28	10:56	27:20	32:48	54:40	5488	10,976
2:46	5:32	11:04	27:40	33:12	55:20	5422	10,843
2:48	5:36	11:12	28:00	33:36	56:00	5357	10,714
2:50	5:40	11:20	28:20	34:00	56:40	5294	10,588
2:52	5:44	11:28	28:40	34:24	57:20	5233	10,465
2:54	5:48	11:36	29:00	34:48	58:00	5172	10,345
2:56	5:52	11:44	29:20	35:12	58:40	5114	10,227
2:58	5:56	11:52	29:40	35:36	59:20	5056	10,112
3:00	6:00	12:00	30:00	36:00	60:00	5000	10,000

In these settings, rowing pace should feel sustainable and repeatable, allowing athletes to transition off the erg without excessive breathlessness or loss of movement quality. A slightly slower split that preserves mechanics and breathing will almost always produce a better overall workout outcome than an aggressive early pace.

The Sprint Start: Launching into the Race!

Feel the surge of adrenaline as you kick off a race with the sprint start — a powerful burst of 8 explosive strokes that set the tone for everything that follows. This is your launch sequence.

The first 6 strokes are pure power: drive hard with your legs and arms, but keep it tight — no layback yet. Think fast, aggressive, and compact. Then, on strokes 7 and 8 add the layback. Pure power of legs, hips and arms. These strokes are short, snappy, and intense — fueled by an energy system that only lasts about 20 seconds. It's a use-it-or-lose-it window. Go beyond 8 strokes and you risk blowing up before you even settle into the race. Done right, it sets up your rhythm; done wrong, it can cost you the whole piece in 15 strokes.

The sprint start is designed for 2000m races or shorter, or the first interval of a workout. It's about creating separation, seizing momentum, and tapping into that raw, anaerobic energy system we all have — but can only use once, at the very start.

CHAPTER 14: PROGRAMMING 101: BUILDING SPEED FOR THE 2K

Effective rowing programming begins with a clear understanding of the 2K, which remains the gold standard for measuring rowing performance. The 2K is not just a test—it is a reference point. Training paces, intensity zones, and workout design all stem from an athlete's current 2K speed. Well-structured programs balance aerobic development, race-pace familiarity, and high-intensity speed while allowing enough volume and recovery to promote consistent progress.

UT2 / Zone 2 (Aerobic Base – Above 2K Pace Steady State)

UT2, also referred to as Zone 2, forms the aerobic foundation of any successful rowing program. This intensity sits well above 2K pace and is designed to be sustainable for long durations. UT2 develops mitochondrial density, stroke efficiency, and cardiovascular capacity while reinforcing technical consistency. These sessions should feel controlled and repeatable. Examples include 3 x 10 minutes with 2–3 minutes of rest or continuous efforts such as 60 minutes of steady-state rowing.

Sprint / Anaerobic Power

Sprint work targets the anaerobic system and focuses on developing peak power, acceleration, and confidence at high speeds. These intervals are short, intense, and require full commitment with adequate recovery. Sprint training teaches athletes how to apply force quickly and maintain technical integrity under maximum output. An example sprint session is 8 x 250 meters with 1 minute of rest, starting at 2K pace and progressively getting faster.

AT / Threshold (Just Above 2K Pace – Middle Distance)

Threshold training, often referred to as AT (Anaerobic Threshold) or lactate threshold work, sits just above 2K pace. This zone is critical for improving an athlete's ability to tolerate discomfort and sustain speed over race-relevant distances. These workouts challenge both aerobic and anaerobic systems and closely mimic the demands of racing. A classic example is 3 x 800 meters with 3 minutes of rest, rowed just faster than 2K pace while maintaining control and rhythm.

Each threshold serves a specific purpose. UT2 builds the engine, threshold training teaches athletes to hold speed under fatigue, and sprint work develops the power needed for starts, moves, and finishes. Effective programming applies these stresses intentionally, using the 2K as the anchor point and progressing systematically over time.

8-Week 2K Pacing Progression
Training by Split, Not Guesswork

After testing your **2000m**, use that split to pace every workout.

Example:
8:00 2K = 2:00/500m
- 2K + 10 → 2:10
- 2K − 2 → 1:58

Slower prescriptions (2K + 16 or more) may feel easy. That's intentional. If you can maintain the assigned **SPM**, you may row slightly faster. Easy means you're fitter — and ready to improve.

Priorities:
Hold the pace • Respect the stroke rate • Be consistent

Week 1

- 2K test (baseline)
- 4×5:00 / 2:00 @ 20-24 − 2K+15
- 12×200m / 1:00 − open − 2K-2
- 3×8:00 / 3:00 → 20spm 2K+18 (2), 22spm 2K+16

Week 2

- 6×400m / 2:00 − 2K pace
- 3×1500m / 2:30 → 22spm +16 | 24spm +14 | 26spm +12
- 10×1:00 / 1:00 − descend from 2K
- 2×12:00 / 3:30 → 20spm +18 | 22spm +16

Week 3

- 3×750m / 4:00 − 2K pace
- 3×9:00 / 2:15 @ 24 − +14
- 12×250m / 1:00 − descend
- 15× :30 on / :30 off − start +3

Week 4

- 6×500m / 2:00 − near 2K
- 5K for time − goal ≤ 2K+10
- 8×2:00 / 2:00 → 1:30 @ +4, :30 sprint −2
- 1000/750/500/250 − 2:30 rest − descend from +7

Week 5

- 1K for time + 10:00 easy @ 24
- 30:00 recovery
- 9×300m / 1:15 — descend
- 3×3:00 @ 26 +12 → rest → 3×2:00 @ 28 +8

Week 6

- 1000/800/600/400/200 — 2:00 rest — descend from +4
- 4×10:00 / 2:00 → 22spm +16 (2), 24spm +14 (2)
- 5×1:30 +3 → rest → 10× :45 -3
- 4×1000m / 2:30 @ 24-28 — descend from +12

Week 7

- 8×500m / 2:00 — near 2K
- 6K recovery
- 500/400/300/200/100/200/300/400/500 — 1:00 rest
- 3×1200m / 2:00 @ 24-28 — +12 or faster

Week 8

- 1333m @ pace → 667m -1 → 333m max
- 4×15:00 / 3:00 @ 20-24 — +20
- 4×500m race pace
- Rest → 2K retest

CHAPTER 15: COMMON FAULTS & CORRECTIONS

FAULT: Early Hip
AKA: Opening the Back Too Early

What You See:
The hips open early in the drive. The shoulders lead before the legs have transferred power.

Why It Matters:
- Power shifts from legs to lower back
- Reduced efficiency and peak force
- Increased fatigue and injury risk

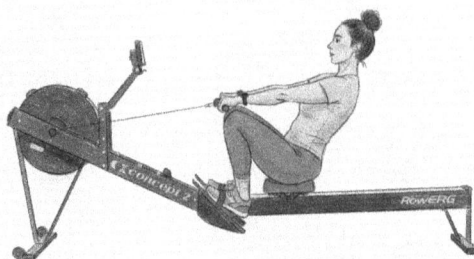

Coach It Fast:
- **Visual**: Demonstrate hips staying back as legs initiate drive
- **Verbal:** Legs before hips. Seat and handle move together. The longer your shoulders stay forward in the drive the better. Use your body like a whip. Look down at the slide during the drive.
- **Tactile / Drill:** Sticky catch. Banded slide

FAULT: Early Knee Bend (Recovery)
AKA: Knees Up Too Soon

What You See:
Knees bend before arms are fully away and the body has pivoted forward during the recovery.

Why It Matters:
- Breaks sequencing
- Causes handle-knee interference
- Arrives at the catch without the body in catch position.
- Rushes the recovery

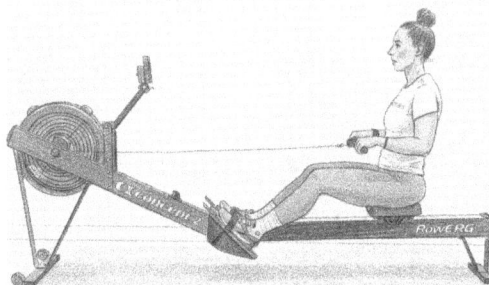

Coach It Fast:
- **Visual:** With legs straight, lean your body forward
- **Verbal:** Hands away, body over, then knees. Keep the legs long until the handle clears. Shoulders over your knees before you bend them on the way back in.
- **Tactile / Drill:** Gentle pressure on the knee/shins while they row and ask them to get the handle to your hand before they go to the catch. Pause drill.

FAULT: Early Arm Bend

What You See:
Arms bend at the catch instead of staying long through the leg drive.

Why It Matters:
- Arms fatigue early
- Leg power never reaches the handle
- Risk of developing tennis/golfer's elbow

Coach It Fast:
- **Visual:** Demonstrate bent elbows at the catch
- **Verbal:** Push, don't pull. If the arms bend, the power ends. Turn your elbows to the floor. Hang from the catch
- **Tactile / Drill:** Sticky catch

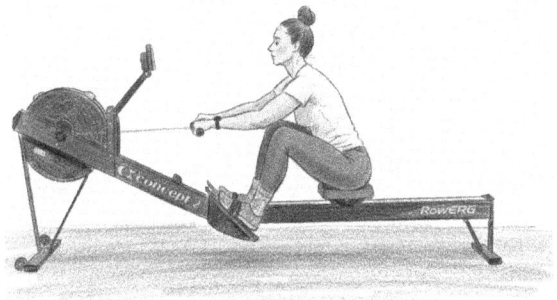

FAULT: Poor Finish

What You See:
Broken wrists, curled handle, missed sternum, shrugged shoulders, or excessive tension.

Why It Matters:
- Reduced efficiency

- Increased shoulder and neck strain

Coach It Fast:
- **Visual:** Tap and release the arms
- **Verbal:** Tap and release. Finish at the sternum. Fast arms away. Relax the arms away. Squeeze your shoulder blades together in that back at the finish. Tap the nipple line.
- **Tactile:** You could touch their middle back and ask them to squeeze there at the finish.

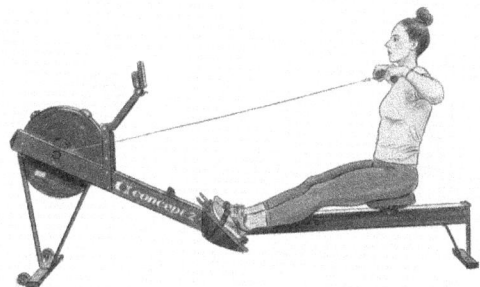

FAULT: Heels Up

What You See:
Athlete drives primarily through the toes, lifting the heels excessively at the catch and through the drive.

Why It Matters:
- Poor connection to the foot stretcher
- Reduced leg drive power
- Often leads to early hip opening, rounding the back and not reaching into the catch.

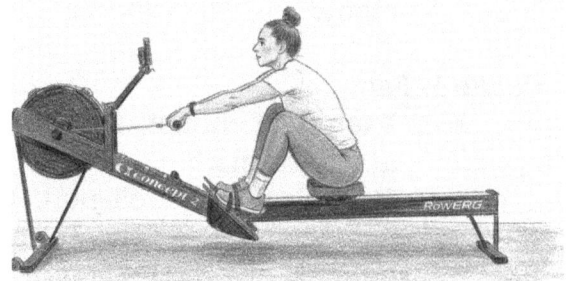

Coach It Fast:
- **Visual:** Point directly to the heels
- **Verbal:** Press through your heels. Heels down.
- **Coach's Note:**
  "Heels down" is a cue, not a rigid rule. A slight heel rise at the catch is acceptable as skill improves, provided pressure stays through the mid-foot and heels. Excessive lift is not. If you give them an inch, they'll take a foot.
- **Tactile / Setup**: Band the slide. Adjust foot stretcher smaller (temporary fix)

FAULT: Poor Chain Path

What You See:
The handle drops, rises, or bounces during the recovery.

Why It Matters:
- Wastes energy
- Disrupts rhythm and efficiency
- Indicates poor connection to the machine

Coach It Fast:
- **Visual:** Demonstrate a wavy chain
- **Verbal:** Straight line from catch to finish. Keep the core engaged during the recovery.
- **Tactile / Drill:** Chalk line or tape marking chain path

FAULT: Rounded Back

What You See:
Collapsed posture with a rounded spine and poor core engagement.

Why It Matters:
- Increased spinal stress
- Reduced force transfer

Coach It Fast:
- **Visual:** Demonstrate tall posture
- **Verbal:** Proud chest, flat back. Brace your core.
- **Tactile / Drill:** No handle no feet drills. Touch the rounded back and ask them to flatten it.

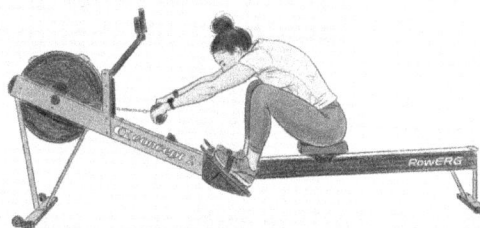

FAULT: Hands-on Handle Placement

What You See:
Incorrect grip: thumbs misplaced, hands too centered, excessive tension.

Why It Matters:
- Poor wrist alignment
- Excess tension
- Shortened stroke length

Coach It Fast:
- **Visual:** Wave fingers to show relaxed grip
- **Verbal:** Thumbs wrapped. Pinkies to the edge. Loose grip like you are holding 2 birds.
- **Tactile / Drill:** Manually adjust hand placement

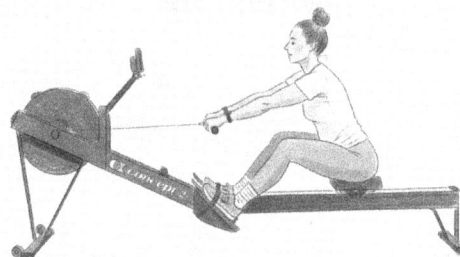

FAULT: Not Completing the Catch

What You See:
Athlete fails to fully reach into the catch position.

Why It Matters:
- Shortened stroke length
- Limited power potential

Coach It Fast:
- **Visual:** Demonstrate full reach
- **Verbal:** Reach ALL the way into the catch. Long is strong.
- **Tactile / Drill:** Tape or chalk line at the catch. Tap the line as a reference.

FAULT: Pulling Into the Catch

What You See:
Athlete pulls themselves forward using the foot straps instead of controlling the recovery.

Why It Matters:
- Loss of control/connection
- Poor positioning at the catch
- Increased hip flexor strain and injury risk

Coach It Fast:
- **Visual**: Point to the toes
- **Verbal:** Push the toes into the foot stretcher at the finish and through the recovery.
- **Tactile / Drill:** Strapless rowing

FAULT: Poor Seated Position
AKA: Pooping Dog

What You See:
Posterior pelvic tilt, rounded back, collapsed posture on the seat.

Why It Matters:
- Destroys posture and power transfer
- Prevents proper catch position
- Often leads to early hip fault
- The body can not pivot freely at the hip if you are sitting on your spine.

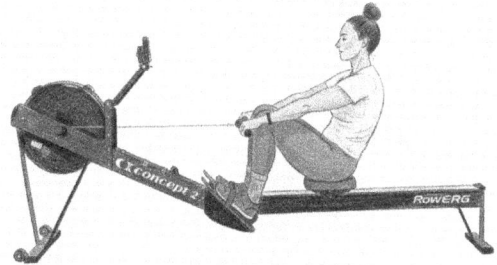

Coach It Fast:
- **Visual:** Demonstrate incorrect sitting posture
- **Verbal:** Sit on your hip bones. "Off the butthole" Feel your hamstrings on the seat.

FAULT: Shooting the Slide
AKA:Taco Shell/ Legs Drive Without the Body

What You See:
Legs extend quickly while the torso stays forward and the handle lags behind.

Why It Matters:
- Leg power is wasted
- Increased risk of back injury

Coach It Fast:
- **Visual**: Demonstrate folding torso
- **Verbal:** Legs and body together. Chest up. Don't change your hip angle as you drive back the seat. Engage the core as you push the seat back.
- **Tactile / Drill:** Raise the monitor. Hold a hand above the screen as a posture cue. "Look up here as you drive back"

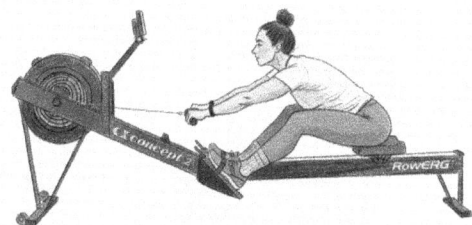

FAULT: Handle Drop at the Catch
AKA: The Waterfall

What You See:
The handle drops after passing the knees on
the recovery.

Why It Matters:
- Breaks rhythm
- Disrupts chain control
- Leads to bad catch position

Coach It Fast:
- **Visual**: Mark a straight return
  path with chalk or tape
- **Verbal:** Guide the chain back
  straight. Don't drop the handle past the knees.
- **Tactile / Drill:** Hold hands under the chain.

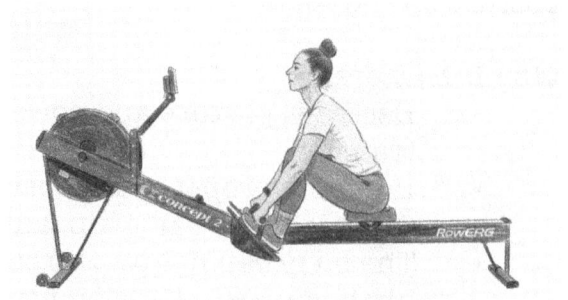

FAULT: Crashing Into the Catch
AKA: Excessive Forward Lean / Over-Reach

What You See:
Athlete rushes into the catch and collapses the chest forward.

Why It Matters:
- Weak, unsupported position
- Compromised drive
- Increased risk of back injury

Coach It Fast:
- **Visual:** Demonstrate crashing motion
- **Verbal:** Smooth into the catch.
- **Tactile / Drill:** Tiny circles drill. Raise the monitor and cue eyes forward

FAULT: Pausing on the Recovery

What You See:
Athlete stops the flywheel at the body or after arms away.

Why It Matters:
- Kills rhythm
- Loses flywheel momentum

Coach It Fast:
- **Visual**: Demonstrate pause
- **Verbal:** Smooth recovery. Don't rest the handle on your leg during the recovery.
- **Tactile / Drill:** One Pause drill (arms away : stroke)

FAULT: Weak Drive

What You See:
Broken or inconsistent power application during the drive.

Why It Matters:
- Limited force production

Coach It Fast:
- **Visual:** Show the force curve
- **Verbal:** Brace your core and PUSH.

FAULT: Seat Hits the Feet

What You See:
Seat crashes into the heels at the catch.

Why It Matters:
- Indicates loss of control
- Usually linked to poor posture and/ or early knee bend

Coach It Fast:
- **Visual:** Demonstrate crashing at the bottom of a squat
- **Verbal:** Control the slide. Heels down into the catch.
- **Tactile / Drill:** Pause drill. Strapless rowing. Band the slide. Put their cell phone on the slide and tell them not to hit it.

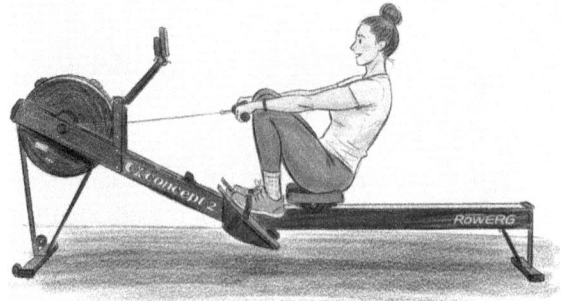

FAULT: Excessive Layback
AKA: Over-Finishing the Stroke

What You See:
Athlete leans too far back and pulls the handle toward the chin.

Why It Matters:
- Increased neck and lower-back strain
- Reduced efficiency

Coach It Fast:
- **Visual:** PVC pipe at 12 o'clock
- **Verbal:** Cut the layback. Finish at 12 o'clock.
- **Tactile / Drill:** Touch back at 1 o'clock and say "that's it, you don't need to go further than that"

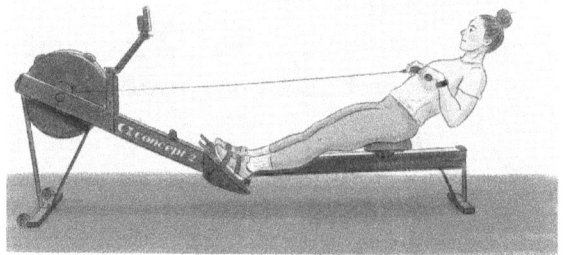

CHAPTER 16: STROKE MECHANICS AND FEEDBACK TOOLS

Using the Force Curve as a Coaching Tool

The force curve on the Concept2 Rower is one of the most effective tools for teaching and refining stroke mechanics. Displayed on the monitor during each stroke, the curve represents how force is applied throughout the drive phase—from catch to finish. A smooth, bell-shaped curve indicates that power is being applied in a consistent, connected sequence: legs first, then the body, then the arms.

As a coach, this visual allows you to connect technical instruction with real-time feedback. If the curve shows a sharp spike, a flat start, or an early drop-off, it's a sign that something in the stroke is off—perhaps an early arm pull, a lack of leg drive, or disconnection through the body. These irregularities become visible and correctable on the screen.

Coaching cues like "push through the legs," "hang with the lats," and "finish clean with the arms" can be paired with force curve feedback to help athletes understand not just what to do, but how it should feel. Over time, they begin to link a smooth force curve with an efficient, powerful stroke—developing both technique and awareness.

Encouraging athletes to occasionally row in "force curve mode" helps reinforce good habits, spot inefficiencies, and build a deeper connection between movement and output. It's not just a display—it's a teaching tool.

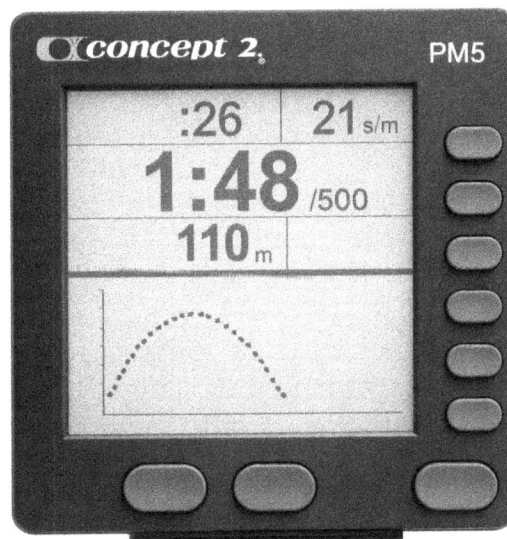

Dynamic Training with Concept2 Slides — Nature's Form Corrector

One of the most underutilized yet highly effective tools in indoor rowing training is the Concept2 Slide system. By placing the rowing machine on a set of slides—small platforms with rollers—you transform the static erg into a dynamic training machine that more closely mimics the feel of rowing on the water.

When rowing on a static erg, the rower moves back and forth while the machine stays anchored. This often leads to form flaws such as early layback, or rushing the recovery. The Slide system shifts this dynamic. When placed on slides, the machine is free to move in response to the rower's motion. This encourages a more natural stroke rhythm, smoother transitions, and proper body mechanics. It punishes poor timing and rewards clean, efficient strokes—hence, the nickname: Nature's Form Corrector.

Key Benefits:

Improves Timing and Connection: The movement of the machine demands precise coordination. The rower must connect legs, hips, and arms in sync to generate momentum.

Enhances Water Feel: The dynamic motion is closer to the experience of rowing in a shell, making it an excellent tool for bridging the gap between erg work and on-water performance.

Promotes Smooth Recovery: Any jerky or rushed movements are exaggerated on the slides, teaching athletes to stay patient and composed during the recovery.

Feel the leg drive: People describe the drive like a leg press machine on the slides.

Builds Boat Sense: Multiple ergs can be linked together on slides, allowing athletes to match stroke rate and rhythm as a crew—perfect for timing drills.

How to Use Slides Effectively:

Start with short technical pieces to let the rower feel how the machine responds to subtle changes in form.
Progress to steady-state rowing, focusing on consistency and rhythm.
Use team-link setups for stroke rate challenges, relay workouts, or practice starts as a crew.

Whether you're coaching novices or tuning up competitive rowers, the Concept2 Slides are an invaluable addition to your toolkit. They don't just make the erg feel more like a boat—they teach your athletes how to move like rowers.

CHAPTER 17: THE UNDERGROUND WORLD OF INDOOR RACING

Beyond the gym and beyond the erg is a global community of indoor racers—a tight-knit, gritty, and passionate group that thrives both in packed race halls and behind screens around the world. While indoor racing has long been associated with the winter months, this underground world is very much alive year-round.

From high-stakes, in-person events like CRASH-B Sprints in Boston, Erg Sprints, the World Rowing Indoor Championships, the Versa Challenge, and regional indoor championships across the country, athletes of all levels come together to test themselves. Olympic rowers line up next to weekend warriors, masters athletes race alongside high school novices, and garage grinders—athletes training alone in basements and spare rooms—earn their place on the leaderboard. Indoors, everyone starts equal. Same machine. Same distance. Same truth. But the heart of indoor racing doesn't live only on race day. It lives online.

Through virtual platforms, online leagues, and remote competitions, indoor racers connect across time zones and continents. Athletes who may never meet in person become training partners, rivals, and friends. Online competitions and ranking systems allow rowers to compare results, chase personal bests, and stack themselves against others who share the same obsession with improvement. What starts as a solo training session often turns into a shared pursuit—linked by splits, screenshots, and results uploaded from thousands of miles apart. This is a community built on effort, honesty, and respect for the work. There are no shortcuts indoors. No water conditions to blame. No steering mistakes. No excuses. Just you, the machine, and the numbers. Indoor racing strips the sport down to its most raw and revealing form, and that shared suffering creates a bond that's hard to replicate elsewhere.

Many indoor racers train primarily—or exclusively—on the Concept2 rowing machine. For them, the erg isn't just a tool for the offseason; it's the arena. It's where seasons are built, identities are formed, and goals are chased year after year. Whether racing a 2K, a sprint, a marathon, or a team relay, these athletes return again and again for the same reason: to see what they're capable of when nothing is hidden.

Indoor racing may exist outside the spotlight, but it is anything but small. It's global. It's relentless. And once you step into it, you're never really training alone again.

CHAPTER 18: WHY ROWING IS THE ULTIMATE ENDURANCE SPORT

Rowing is the ultimate endurance sport because it demands sustained power from the entire body, not just the lungs or the legs. Unlike running or cycling, rowing requires continuous coordination between the legs, hips, trunk, and arms while maintaining precise sequencing under fatigue. As effort increases, there is nowhere to hide—poor technique, weak links, and inefficient movement are exposed immediately. Endurance in rowing is not just about lasting longer; it is about repeatedly applying force with control, rhythm, and efficiency over thousands of strokes. This combination of aerobic capacity, muscular endurance, technical discipline, and mental resilience is what separates rowing from other endurance modalities—and why it produces athletes who are not just fit, but durable.

Zone 2 Training (UT2): Building the Aerobic Engine

Zone 2 training—often referred to in rowing as UT2—is the foundation of long-term endurance development. It represents low-intensity, sustainable work that can be maintained for extended periods while remaining primarily aerobic. Although it may not feel as challenging as high-intensity training, UT2 is where the majority of aerobic adaptations occur and where durable endurance is built.

In rowing, UT2 is typically performed at lower stroke rates with controlled power output, emphasizing efficiency, rhythm, and technical precision. This training zone allows athletes to accumulate meaningful volume without excessive fatigue, making it a cornerstone of successful rowing programs at every level.

Why Zone 2 (UT2) Matters

UT2 training improves the body's ability to produce energy aerobically. Over time, consistent work in this zone leads to increased mitochondrial density, improved fat utilization, and enhanced oxygen delivery to working muscles. These adaptations allow athletes to row harder for longer while delaying fatigue.

Zone 2 training also supports recovery. Because it places minimal stress on the nervous system and musculoskeletal system, UT2 can be performed frequently without compromising performance in harder sessions. This makes it ideal for building weekly volume, reinforcing technique, and maintaining consistency throughout a season.

Key benefits of Zone 2 (UT2) training include:

• Improved aerobic base and endurance

• Increased efficiency and stroke economy

- Enhanced fat metabolism

- Lower injury risk compared to high-intensity work

- Faster recovery between hard training sessions

- Long-term cardiovascular health

Why Rowing Is Superior for Zone 2 Training
Rowing is uniquely suited for Zone 2 training because it engages the entire body in a rhythmic, repeatable motion. Unlike many endurance modalities that emphasize only the lower body, rowing distributes work across the legs, trunk, and upper body, allowing athletes to sustain steady output without overloading a single area.

The rowing machine also provides immediate, objective feedback. Stroke rate, split, heart rate, and perceived effort can be monitored in real time, allowing athletes to stay precisely within the UT2 zone. This level of control makes rowing one of the most accurate tools available for aerobic development.

Additionally, rowing at UT2 intensities reinforces sound technique. Lower stroke rates and manageable power outputs allow athletes to focus on sequencing, posture, and efficiency—habits that carry over directly to higher-intensity work and racing.

What Zone 2 (UT2) Should Feel Like
Zone 2 rowing should feel sustainable and controlled. Athletes should be able to breathe rhythmically, maintain good posture, and hold conversation in short phrases. Effort should feel steady rather than strained, with no burning in the legs and no loss of technical control.

The goal of UT2 is not to chase speed, but to accumulate quality work. Discipline in this zone is critical. Athletes who row UT2 too hard often undermine its benefits, turning aerobic work into something it was never intended to be.

The Long-Term Payoff
Zone 2 training may not be flashy, but it is powerful. It builds the aerobic engine that supports every hard piece, every race, and every season of development. Athletes who commit to UT2 consistently move better, recover faster, and sustain higher performance over time.

In rowing, speed is built on endurance, and endurance is developed through Zone 2 work. This type of training is commonly called long slow distance (LSD), but at its core it is about accumulating meaningful time under tension.
16–19

CHAPTER 19: THE COLLEGIATE RECRUITING PROCESS

Opportunity, Standards, and What Coaches Are Really Looking For
For high school rowers, the collegiate recruiting process represents one of the greatest opportunities in sport. Rowing is unique: it rewards long-term development, discipline, teamwork, and grit just as much as raw talent. For athletes willing to commit to the process, rowing can open doors to elite universities, financial support, and life-changing educational opportunities.

The Benchmark: Why the International Standard Matters
At the highest levels, collegiate rowing programs measure athletes against international standards. These systems set the benchmark for technical proficiency, work capacity, and mental toughness. College coaches recruit athletes who show the potential to meet these standards, even if they are not fully developed yet. Recruiting is not only about where an athlete is today, but about how fast they are improving.
Progress matters. Coaches track:

- Year-over-year improvement

- Responsiveness to training

- Technical growth

- The ability to handle increasing training loads

Athletes who demonstrate steady upward trajectories often recruit better than those who peak early.

What College Coaches Are Looking For
While performance metrics matter, collegiate level coaches are building programs, not just boats. They are evaluating the whole athlete.

1. Performance and Potential
Yes, erg scores matter—especially the 2K—but they are not viewed in isolation. Coaches want to know:

- How long has this athlete been rowing?

- How fast are they improving?

- Are they durable and trainable?

- Do they move well and stay healthy?

An excellent 2K paired with technical competence and physical durability makes an athlete highly recruitable.

2. Coachability
Coachability is one of the most valuable traits in the recruiting process.
Coaches look for athletes who:

- Listen and apply feedback quickly

- Can adjust technique under pressure

- Take responsibility for mistakes

- Trust the training process rather than fighting it

Highly coachable athletes adapt faster in collegiate programs, and coaches know this.

3. Grit and Work Ethic
Grit and work ethic are non-negotiable. Rowing is demanding, and college programs train early, often, and with intensity. Coaches want athletes who show up consistently, push through discomfort, respond to adversity with effort instead of excuses, and compete daily, not just on race day. Grit is often the deciding factor between athletes with similar performance metrics.

- Show up consistently

- Push through discomfort not injury

- Respond to adversity with effort, not excuses

- Compete daily, not just on race day

Grit is often the deciding factor between athletes with similar erg scores.

4. Character
Team culture and character matter. College rowing is a team sport in the truest sense. College rowing is deeply team oriented.
Coaches are recruiting athletes who:

- Support teammates

- Contribute positively

- Handle pressure with maturity

- Lead through actions, not ego

- An athlete who makes everyone around them better is invaluable.

50

Scholarships, Title IX, and Opportunity—Especially for Women

Rowing provides extraordinary opportunity for female athletes.

Due to Title IX, women's D1 rowing is one of the most heavily supported collegiate sports in terms of roster size and scholarship availability. This has created:

- More scholarship opportunities

- Larger team rosters

- Increased access to elite universities

For girls who have the talent, the work ethic, and the personality, rowing can provide financial support and educational access that would be difficult to achieve through academics alone.

This is one of the greatest—and still underutilized—pathways for young women in sport.

Rowing as an Academic Gateway

Rowing is also one of the few sports where performance can significantly impact admissions outcomes, particularly at highly selective institutions.

For both boys and girls:

- A strong 2K

- Consistent training history

- Demonstrated commitment

- Strong coach recommendations

Together, these factors can help athletes gain admission to academically elite schools—including Ivy League institutions—that might otherwise be out of reach. It's important to be clear: rowing does not replace academic performance—it complements it. Strong grades are still required. Rowing may help set a student apart in the admissions process, but it only does so when paired with solid academic achievement. In reality, many successful rowers are strong students already, likely because the sport demands discipline, time management, accountability, and consistency. The same habits that produce a good 2K also tend to produce good grades. Colleges are not choosing between academics and athletics—they are looking for students who demonstrate excellence in both.

Rowing rewards students who excel in discipline, persistence, and execution.

The recruiting process is not about shortcuts.
It is about:

• Building strong, durable athletes

• Developing technical proficiency

• Showing consistent progress

• Becoming someone a coach wants in their program for four years

When athletes commit to this standard—physically, mentally, and culturally—the opportunities are real and abundant. While the academic opportunities created through rowing are very real, the true prize is not simply using the sport as a means to an end. The real achievement is earning the opportunity to row at the collegiate level itself. Student-athletes should view this not as rowing getting them somewhere else, but as rowing bringing them somewhere extraordinary—an environment where they can continue to pursue the sport they love, train at a high level, and be part of a team that values discipline, commitment, and growth. The education is important, but so is the privilege of continuing to row while earning it.

Rowing does not just recruit speed.
It recruits potential, character, and commitment.

Job Opportunities for Collegiate Rowers

Collegiate rowers are highly sought after in the workforce because the demands of the sport closely mirror the traits employers value most. Rowers are trained to manage time effectively, balancing early mornings, rigorous training schedules, academics, and team responsibilities. They are accustomed to accountability, showing up prepared, and performing under pressure. The discipline required to train consistently over multiple years translates directly to reliability and strong work ethic in professional settings.

Rowers also develop exceptional teamwork and communication skills. Success in rowing depends on synchronization, trust, and collective effort—qualities that make rowers effective collaborators and leaders in the workplace. Employers recognize that collegiate rowers are coachable, goal-oriented, and resilient. They know how to receive feedback, adapt quickly, and persist through challenges. As a result, collegiate rowers are often hired first—not simply because they were athletes, but because the sport has prepared them to operate at a high standard long after their rowing careers end.

CHAPTER 20: PSYCHOLOGY & CREATIVITY WITH THE RESISTANT ATHLETE

Every coach will eventually encounter the resistant customer—the one who doesn't seem to want to learn, doesn't respond to cues, and maybe even rolls their eyes during class or practice. It's easy to write them off or assume they just don't care. But in my experience, that's almost never the case.

More often than not, resistant athletes are carrying something heavier than a dumbbell. It could be stress from work, trouble at home, anxiety about being in a gym, or past experiences that made them feel like fitness just isn't for them. That's why the job of a coach—especially in rowing, where form, rhythm, and mindset are deeply intertwined—is to go beyond the surface.

Be relentless in your effort to coach them. If standard cues don't land, get creative. Don't just repeat the same words louder. Reframe. Rephrase. Paint a different picture. Sometimes the key isn't in what you say—it's in when and where you say it. Talk to them after class. Catch them before warm-ups. Ask questions. Be curious about who they are, not just how they move. You might learn something that completely changes how you coach them.

And if they truly don't want to dive deep into technique, that's okay too. Your job is to keep them safe and engaged. Find a baseline of movement that honors their level of athleticism and your standard for quality. Communicate that clearly. Show them you're in this together, and that you're not giving up on them.

In my experience, most of these athletes do want to learn. They want to do it the right way—they just need a teacher who can meet them where they are, believe in their potential, and help guide them to the level of fitness they deserve.

Rowing isn't just a technical skill—it's a teaching opportunity. And the resistant athlete? They're not your hardest student. They're your most important one.

CHAPTER 21: ROWING ETIQUETTE

Respect for the equipment and your teammates is a key part of being a great rower. Practicing proper rowing etiquette helps maintain the longevity of the equipment, ensures a clean and safe training environment, and reflects the discipline expected in the sport.

Control the Handle – Never Let It Slam into the Flywheel.
Always keep control of the handle throughout the workout, especially at the end of a piece. Letting the handle fly forward into the flywheel can damage the machine.

Use the Quick Release Properly
After rowing, release your feet using the quick-release tabs on the foot stretchers—not by pulling and stretching the black straps. Repeatedly pulling on the straps weakens the strap mechanics and leads to unnecessary wear and tear.

Wipe Down After Use Maintaining Equipment
Understand the importance of storing and cleaning rowing machines to ensure their longevity and performance.
After each session, clean the following areas with a wet wipe.
Handle – Where your hands made contact
Seat – Where you sat
Slide Rails – Where the seat rolls
A clean erg is a shared courtesy.
NEVER WET THE MONITOR.

Rowing is a team sport—even when you're on an erg. Respect for the equipment and your teammates is just as important as the workout itself. Store the handle inside of the flywheel housing. There is a bungee cord on the opposite side. If the handle is always extended, the bungee cord will need replacing. Store the monitor up next to the flywheel housing to protect it when not in use or when moving the machine.

FREQUENTLY ASKED QUESTIONS (FAQ)

What should the damper setting be?
Short answer: Most rowers should start around damper 3-5, not 10.
Reference: See Chapter 12: Drag Factor — explains why damper setting is not resistance, how drag factor works, and why elite rowers use lower settings to reinforce clean sequencing and a strong catch.

How long should I row when I'm starting out?
Short answer: Start with short segments (2-5 minutes) and build gradually.
Reference: See Chapter 18 (Zone 2 / UT2 Training) — explains how aerobic development is built through sustainable volume, not early exhaustion.

What stroke rate should I row at?
Short answer: Row at a rate you can control, usually 20-28 SPM for most training.
Reference: See Chapter 11: Using the Rowing Monitor — stroke rate reflects recovery speed, not effort. Power comes from force per stroke, not higher rates.

Does a higher stroke rate mean I'm working harder?
Short answer: No. Higher rate does not equal higher effort.
Reference: See Chapter 11 (Watts, Stroke Output, and Consistency) — watts and force curve reveal real work; stroke rate only shows how fast you're moving.

How often should I row?
Short answer: Most people benefit from rowing every other day or 3-5x per week.
Reference: See Chapter 18: Zone 2 Training — explains how rowing supports frequent training when intensity and technique are managed correctly.

Does lifting weights help rowing?
Short answer: Yes. Strength training protects rowers and improves power.
Reference: See Chapter 6: Strength Training for Injury Prevention — outlines key lifts that build the posterior chain, core stability, and shoulder resilience.

What's the difference between aerobic and anaerobic rowing?
Short answer: Aerobic rowing is sustainable and conversational. Anaerobic rowing is short, hard, and uncomfortable.
Reference: See Chapters 13 — explains UT2, threshold, sprint work, and how each energy system fits into smart programming.

What's the best strategy for racing a 2000m?
Short answer: Controlled start, honest middle, strong finish.
Reference: See Chapter 13: Racing the 2K — covers pacing strategy, sprint start, negative splitting, and mental execution.

Why do my forearms tighten up when I row?
Short answer: You're likely bending the arms early or gripping too tightly.
Reference: See Chapter 15: Common Faults — Early Arm Bend & Grip Errors — includes drills and cues to transfer work back to the legs and lats.

How do I stop the seat from hitting my heels?
Short answer: Hands and body move first. Knees come last.
Reference: See Chapter 2: The Recovery and Chapter 15: Early Knee Bend — sequencing errors on the recovery cause loss of control at the catch.

Why does rowing bother my back?
Short answer: Rowing hurts backs when hips aren't doing their job.
Reference: See Chapter 8: Common Rowing Injuries and Chapter 6: Strength Training — explains why hip strength, posture, and sequencing protect the spine.

Is rowing safe for older adults?
Short answer: Yes — when taught correctly, rowing is one of the safest full-body modalities available.
Reference: See Chapter 1: The Science Behind the Stroke — reviews research showing rowing improves cardiovascular fitness and power in older populations without increased injury risk.

Final Coaching Reminder
Rowing problems are rarely solved by rowing harder.
They are solved by better sequencing, better positions, and better standards.

This book exists to make those standards clear.

ROWING GLOSSARY: COMMON TERMINOLOGY

2K (2000 Meter Test)
The standard benchmark test in rowing. Used to measure performance, set training paces, and evaluate progress. Central to collegiate recruiting and program design.

Anaerobic
Energy production that occurs without sufficient oxygen. Used during high-intensity efforts such as sprints and race finishes.

Anaerobic Threshold (AT)
The intensity at which lactate begins to accumulate faster than it can be cleared. Often trained just above 2K pace. Critical for improving race performance.

Arms Away
The first movement of the recovery, where the arms extend forward from the finish before the body pivots or the knees bend.

Biofeedback
Information displayed on the Performance Monitor that reflects effort and output, such as pace, watts, heart rate, and stroke rate.

Body Over
The phase of the recovery where the torso pivots forward from the hips after the arms extend and before the knees bend.

Catch
The position where the seat and handle are closest to the flywheel. This marks the start of the drive. On the water, it is when the oar enters the water.

Chain Path
The straight-line path the handle should travel from the catch to the finish and back. Efficient rowing requires a smooth, level chain path.

Cooldown
A period of low-intensity rowing after training that helps the body transition toward recovery and reduces stiffness.

Damper Setting
The numbered lever on the flywheel housing that controls airflow. Higher settings allow more air in and feel heavier. Lower settings simulate a lighter, faster boat.

Drag Factor
A numerical value calculated by the monitor that reflects actual resistance felt, independent of damper setting. Used for precise setup.

Drive
The power phase of the stroke. Sequence: legs push first, followed by the body swing, finishing with the arms.

Ergometer (Erg)
A device that measures work. The indoor rowing machine is commonly referred to as an erg.

Finish
The position at the end of the drive where the handle is drawn to the body and the torso leans back slightly. On the water, this is when the oar exits the water.

Flexfoot
The adjustable foot stretcher that secures the feet during rowing.

Force Curve
A graphical display on the monitor showing how power is applied throughout the stroke. Used to assess efficiency and timing.

Forward Body Angle
A hinged position from the hips with the torso leaning forward, used at the catch to prepare for leg drive.

Heart Rate (HR)
Beats per minute (BPM) reflecting cardiovascular response. Used to monitor intensity zones such as UT2 or threshold.

Hypercompression (Overcompression)
Excessive knee bend at the catch where the seat comes too close to the heels, typically past vertical shins. Reduces power and stability.

Interval
A structured workout consisting of alternating work and rest periods, based on time or distance.

Layback
The backward lean of the torso at the finish. Ideally 5–10 degrees from vertical.

Leg Drive
The initial and primary source of power in the stroke, generated by pushing through the legs.

Load
The resistance felt during the drive, influenced by drag factor, stroke power, and technique.

Meters
The distance unit displayed on the monitor, calculated from power output rather than actual movement.

Monorail
The track on which the seat slides.

Negative Splits
A pacing strategy where speed increases progressively throughout a workout or race.

Pace
The time it takes to row 500 meters, shown as time/500m. Lower numbers indicate faster speed.

Paddling
Very low-intensity rowing used for recovery or between pieces.

Piece
A defined segment of rowing work measured by time or distance.

PM5 (Performance Monitor)
The computer attached to the erg that displays performance data including pace, stroke rate, watts, and heart rate.

Power Curve
Another term for force curve, showing how effectively force is applied during the stroke.

Ratio
The relationship between drive time and recovery time. Efficient rowing emphasizes a longer recovery than drive.

Recovery
The relaxed phase of the stroke moving from finish back to catch. Sequence: arms, body, then legs.

Rest
A period of complete rest or low-intensity movement between intervals or pieces.

Rolling Start
Beginning the next interval while already moving, typically entering the next piece with 10 seconds remaining in rest.

Sequence
The correct order of movements during the stroke.
Drive: Legs → Body → Arms
Recovery: Arms → Body → Legs

Split
The displayed pace at any moment, typically shown as time per 500 meters.

SPM (Strokes Per Minute)
The number of complete strokes taken per minute.

Steady State
Continuous rowing at a controlled intensity, usually within UT2 or UT1 zones.

Stroke Rate
Another term for SPM, indicating how fast strokes are being taken.

Swing
The smooth pivot of the torso from forward body angle to layback during the drive.

Threshold Training
Training performed near or slightly above anaerobic threshold to improve race endurance.

UT2 (Utilization Training 2)
Low-intensity aerobic training zone, also known as Zone 2. Used to build endurance, efficiency, and aerobic capacity.

UT1 (Utilization Training 1)
Moderate aerobic intensity above UT2 but below threshold. More demanding but still sustainable.

Warm-Up
Gradual rowing performed before training to increase temperature, mobility, and readiness.

Watts
A direct measurement of power output displayed on the monitor.

Work
The effort-focused portion of a workout.

Work Output

The measurable result of effort, shown as pace, watts, or calories on the Performance Monitor.

Zone 2

Another term for UT2. Aerobic endurance training zone that supports long-term performance and recovery.

REFERENCES

1 Concept2 Rowing Handbook. "The Rowing Stroke." Concept2 Inc.
(Referenced in sections discussing stroke sequence, leg drive initiation, and body swing.)

2 Concept2 Rowing Handbook. "Force Curve and Power Application." Concept2 Inc.
(Referenced in sections explaining force transfer, timing, and efficiency.)

3 Concept2 Rowing Handbook. "Drag Factor vs. Damper Setting." Concept2 Inc.
(Referenced in sections discussing resistance, load, and erg setup.)

4 Concept2 Rowing Handbook. "Understanding Pace, Watts, and Meters." Concept2 Inc.
(Referenced in sections covering performance metrics and biofeedback.)

5 Concept2 Rowing Handbook. "Training Intensity Zones." Concept2 Inc.
(Referenced in UT2, threshold, and programming sections.)

Expanded References – Scientific Studies on Rowing

Comparative Physiology, Energy Cost, and Exercise Intensity

6 Gilligan, W. E., Bezoni, J., & Webster, M. J. (1984).
A comparison of the physiological responses to rowing and cycling exercise using ratings of perceived exertion as an indicator of exercise intensity.
Poster presentation, American College of Sports Medicine Conference, 1984.

7 Hagerman, F. C., & Mansfield, M. C. (1988).
A comparison of energy cost and mechanical efficiency at identical power outputs between a mechanically variable-resistance rowing ergometer and a mechanically fixed-resistance bicycle ergometer.
Medicine & Science in Sports & Exercise, 20(5), 479–488.

8 Mahler, D. A., Andrea, B. E., & Ward, J. L. (1987).
Comparison of exercise performance on rowing and cycle ergometers.
Research Quarterly for Exercise and Sport, 58(4), 341–346.

9 Zeni, A. I., Hoffman, M. D., & Clifford, P. S. (1996).
Energy expenditure with indoor exercise machines.
Journal of the American Medical Association (JAMA), 275(18), 1424–1427.

Rowing Physiology, Oxygen Uptake, and Aerobic Capacity

10 DiPrampero, P. E., Cortili, G., Celentano, F., & Cerretelli, P. (1971).
Physiological aspects of rowing.
Journal of Applied Physiology, 31(6), 853-857.

11 Hagerman, F. C., Connors, M. C., Gault, J. A., Hagerman, G. R., & Polinski, W. J.
(1978).
Energy expenditure during simulated rowing.
Journal of Applied Physiology, 45(1), 87-93.

12 Hagerman, F. C. (1984).
Applied physiology of rowing.
Sports Medicine, 1(4), 303-326.

13 Hagerman, F. C., & Lee, W. D. (1971).
Measurement of oxygen consumption, heart rate, and work output during rowing.
Medicine & Science in Sports, 3(4), 155-160.

14 Ishiko, T. (1967).
Aerobic capacity and external criteria of performance.
Journal of the Canadian Medical Association, 96, 746-749.

15 Jackson, R. C., & Secher, N. H. (1976).
The aerobic demands of rowing in two Olympic rowers.
Medicine & Science in Sports, 8(3), 168-170.

16 Lakomy, H. K. A., & Lakomy, J. (1993).
Estimation of maximum oxygen uptake from submaximal exercise on a Concept2
rowing ergometer.
Journal of Sports Sciences, 11, 227-232.

Rowing and Aging / Clinical Populations

17 Mark, S., Hagerman, F. C., Falkel, J. E., Murray, T. F., & Ragg, K. E. (1993).
Rowing and cycle ergometer exercise in the elderly.
Journal of Sports Sciences, 11, 227-232.

18 Hagerman, F. C., et al. (1996).
A 20-year longitudinal study of Olympic oarsmen.
Medicine & Science in Sports & Exercise, 28(8), 1150-1156.
Technique, Kinesiology, and Instructional Foundations

19 Mazzone, T. (1988).
Kinesiology of the rowing stroke.
NSCA Journal, 10(2).

20 Mazzone, T. (1988).
Kinesiology of the rowing stroke.
NSCA Journal, 10(2).

21 Brown, B. (1986).
Stroke! A Guide to Recreational Rowing.
Camden, ME: International Marine Publishing Company.

22 Churbuck, D. C. (1988).
The Book of Rowing.
Woodstock, VT: The Overlook Press.

23 Kirch, B., Hoyt, R., & Fithian, J. (1985).
Row for Your Life.
New York, NY: Simon & Schuster.

24 Mendenhall, T. (1980).
A Short History of American Rowing.
Boston, MA: Charles River Books.

Environmental & Performance Factors

25 Peltonen, J., et al. (1994).
Effects of oxygen fraction in inspired air on rowing performance.
Medicine & Science in Sports & Exercise, 26, 573-579.

26 Stuller, J. (1986).
Terrestrial rowing.
Physician and Sportsmedicine, 14(3), 272-276.

About the Author

Lizzy Carson has built her life around one belief: rowing changes lives.

She is the owner of Concept Fitness, a premier rowing and strength training facility on the South Shore of Long Island, and the founder of Concept Crew, a nonprofit program that introduces students to rowing and helps guide them toward collegiate opportunities through sport.

A multiple Concept2 world record holder and 2021 CrossFit Games athlete, Lizzy combines elite performance experience with years of hands-on coaching. As a Concept2 Master Instructor, she educates coaches and athletes on proper technique, programming, and sustainable training methods.

Her mission is simple — make rowing accessible, teach it the right way, and help people become stronger, healthier, and more confident through the process.

The Rowing Standard is the culmination of that mission.

www.ingramcontent.com/pod-product-compliance
Lightning Source LLC
Chambersburg PA
CBHW080045280326
41935CB00014B/1790